Study Guide for Foundations of Professional Personal Training

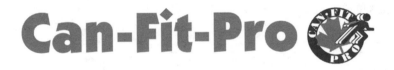

Can-Fit-Pro

Mike Bates

Gregory Anderson

EDITORS

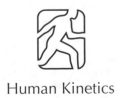

Human Kinetics

ISBN-10: 0-7360-6911-9
ISBN-13: 978-0-7360-6911-3

The Web addresses cited in this text were current as of May 23, 2007, unless otherwise noted.

Acquisitions Editor: Michael S. Bahrke, PhD
Managing Editor: Lee Alexander
Copyeditor: Alisha Jeddeloh
Proofreader: Bethany J. Bentley
Permission Manager: Dalene Reeder
Graphic Designer: Nancy Rasmus
Graphic Artist: Angela K. Snyder
Cover Designer: Gavin Fung
Photographer (cover): Claus Andersen
Art Manager: Kelly Hendren
Illustrator: Alan L. Wilborn
Printer: Versa Press

Printed in the United States of America   10   9   8   7

The paper in this book is certified under a sustainable forestry program.

Human Kinetics
Web site: www.HumanKinetics.com

United States: Human Kinetics
P.O. Box 5076
Champaign, IL 61825-5076
800-747-4457
e-mail: humank@hkusa.com

Canada: Human Kinetics
475 Devonshire Road, Unit 100
Windsor, ON N8Y 2L5
800-465-7301 (in Canada only)
e-mail: info@hkcanada.com

Europe: Human Kinetics
107 Bradford Road
Stanningley
Leeds LS28 6AT, United Kingdom
+44 (0)113 255 5665
e-mail: hk@hkeurope.com

Australia: Human Kinetics
57A Price Avenue
Lower Mitcham, South Australia 5062
08 8372 0999
e-mail: info@hkaustralia.com

New Zealand: Human Kinetics
P.O. Box 80
Torrens Park, South Australia 5062
0800 222 062
e-mail: info@hknewzealand.com

CONTENTS

PART IV   The Professional Personal Trainer

CREDITS

Figure 1, p. xii—Canadian Physical Activity Guide to Healthy Active Living, Health Canada, 1998, http://www.hc-sc.gc.ca/hppb/paguide/pdf/guideEng.pdf ©Reproduced with permission from the Minister of Public Works and Government Services Canada, 2002.

Figure 6, p. 19—Reprinted, by permission, from J.H. Wilmore and D.L. Costill, 2004, *Physiology of sport and exercise,* 3rd ed. (Champaign, IL: Human Kinetics), p. 209.

Figure 7*a*, p. 20—Reprinted, by permission, from J.H. Wilmore and D.L. Costill, 2004, *Physiology of sport and exercise,* 3rd ed. (Champaign, IL: Human Kinetics), p. 245.

Figure 7*b*, p. 20—Reprinted, by permission, from J.H. Wilmore and D.L. Costill, 2004, *Physiology of sport and exercise,* 3rd ed. (Champaign, IL: Human Kinetics), p. 245.

Figure 8*a*, p. 26—Reprinted, by permission, from National Strength and Conditioning Association, 2000, *Essentials of strength training and conditioning,* 2nd ed. (Champaign, IL: Human Kinetics), p. 27.

Figure 8*b*, p. 26—Reprinted, by permission, from National Strength and Conditioning Association, 2000, *Essentials of strength training and conditioning,* 2nd ed. (Champaign, IL: Human Kinetics), p. 27.

Figure 8*c*, p. 26—Reprinted, by permission, from National Strength and Conditioning Association, 2000, *Essentials of strength training and conditioning,* 2nd ed. (Champaign, IL: Human Kinetics), p. 28.

Figure 9*a*, p. 34—Reprinted, by permission, from National Strength and Conditioning Association, 2000, *Essentials of strength training and conditioning,* 2nd ed. (Champaign, IL: Human Kinetics), p. 29.

Figure 9*b*, p. 34—Reprinted, by permission, from National Strength and Conditioning Association, 2000, *Essentials of strength training and conditioning,* 2nd ed. (Champaign, IL: Human Kinetics), p. 29.

INTRODUCTION

Mike Bates, MBA

Founded in 1993, Can-Fit-Pro was established to assist fitness professionals in their quest for ongoing education and continued professionalism. We meet the needs of Canadian fitness professionals and consumers through our professional fitness certification offerings, conference and tradeshow events, fitness education workshops, and diverse membership offerings.

Our Mission

Can-Fit-Pro takes today's fitness professional challenges and creates tomorrow's solutions through increased opportunities for developing ongoing relative knowledge and personal enrichment.

Our Vision

Our vision is to move away from the survival mode of simply meeting basic needs and into a relationship that demonstrates value and excellence. We believe that our growth and education are complete when we are able to provide for all fitness professionals.

Purpose and Goals of Can-Fit-Pro's Certification Program

Launched in 1998, Can-Fit-Pro's certification program was created to provide a nationally recognized fitness certification for creating qualified professionals. Starting with the two programs fundamental to fitness, group fitness instruction and personal training, Can-Fit-Pro's certification programs now include several specialized certifications to meet the increasingly diverse needs of fitness consumers. Led by our network of qualified course instructors and examiners called *PRO Trainers*, Can-Fit-Pro's certification programs are designed to meet the certification needs of all fitness professionals across Canada by being accessible, attainable, and affordable.

Can-Fit-Pro hosts North America's largest fitness professional conference and tradeshow in Toronto in August every year. In addition, we host a series of regional conference events that allow our certified members to keep their practical skills and knowledge up to date. We will continue to expand our conference offerings to provide continuing education opportunities for fitness professionals.

As a Can-Fit-Pro professional member, you will receive discounts on Can-Fit-Pro certification and conference event registration fees, you will receive our bimonthly industry magazine, and you will have access to discounts with many fitness and nonindustry vendors. Thank you for being a part of the leading edge of fitness training in Canada. Together as fitness professionals, we will educate, communicate, and motivate fitness enthusiasts everywhere toward a healthier and more active lifestyle.

Can-Fit-Pro Certification: A Statement of Excellence

Can-Fit-Pro–certified fitness professionals demonstrate commitment to the fitness industry and show a high standard of competency and ability.

As leaders in the future of Canadian fitness, Can-Fit-Pro–certified fitness professionals provide a reliable source of fitness knowledge and safe, effective exercise for all exercisers. This standard of excellence makes Can-Fit-Pro–certified fitness professionals competitive and in high demand for employment across the country.

Continual training shows a dedication to self-improvement and a commitment to providing motivation and information for all participants. Known for quality and enthusiasm, Can-Fit-Pro–certified fitness professionals establish a benchmark for excellence and education in the fitness industry.

Personal Training Specialist Certification

With the tremendous growth of the fitness industry, there is increased opportunity for certified personal trainers. This growth has resulted in a greater need for knowledgeable, mature, and qualified individuals. The fitness profession is continually challenged to maintain consistent, quality leadership and educational programs. The availability of qualified personal trainers helps to standardize the services clubs are able to offer and helps maintain the credibility of the industry as a whole.

The Personal Training Specialist (PTS) certification has been developed to provide the opportunity to become better educated about personal training in a fun, adult learning atmosphere. This program will enhance your confidence and motivation to lead your clients to be active, feel great, and get results!

An important goal of this program is to have a positive impact on the activity level of Canadians. The Canada's *Integrated Pan-Canadian Healthy Living Strategy* sets healthy-living targets and seeks to obtain a 20% increase by 2015 in the proportion of Canadians who

- are physically active,
- eat healthily, and
- are at a healthy body weight.

The target of this initiative, by which requests for government grants for health promotion and disease prevention are measured, sets the stage for a link between allied health professionals and fitness professionals to provide education and services for Canadians who want to increase their physical activity.

From working in a club to starting your own business, the opportunities for certified personal trainers have never been greater. Can-Fit-Pro is proud to be working alongside the Canadian government and several nongovernmental organizations to get Canadians moving toward improved health.

Our Commitment to You

Can-Fit-Pro and our PRO Trainers promise to

1. educate you to learn the skills to provide safe, effective client sessions;

2. motivate you by providing a learning environment that is educational and fun; and

3. communicate with you so that you are directly involved in your own learning process mentally, verbally, and physically.

Your Commitment to Yourself

To become a PTS, you must promise to

1. take responsibility for your own learning, success, and enjoyment;

2. attend and actively participate in the entire certification preparatory course;

3. complete review assignments and projects as required for you to solidify the theoretical concepts and practical concepts you are learning;

4. network with others to share feedback about this experience and gather information;

5. set realistic goals for yourself so that you meet your deadlines for certification completion;

6. ask questions if you do not understand a concept; and

7. give your best effort both physically and mentally.

Goals and Expectations

For this course of study to be successful, you should outline your expectations and goals for achievement. The following sections will help you with this.

Personal Gains

I am taking this course of study to be able to do the following:

1. _____
   _____

2. _____
   _____

3. _____
   _____

Client Gains

I will provide the following things to clients as a certified PTS:

1. _____
   _____

2. _____
   _____

3. _____
   _____

What You Need to Become Certified

Eligibility

Certification as a Can-Fit-Pro PTS is open to all candidates. Candidates must hold a current cardiopulmonary resuscitation (CPR) certificate.

Recommendations

In order to improve your chances for successful certification, we recommend that you prepare for the theory and practical certification exams by attending the PTS preparatory course. The course will help clarify the theory and practical requirements necessary to be a successful personal trainer and will prepare you for the exams.

To ensure that you are aware of the key theoretical and practical concepts being examined, we recommend that you purchase a copy of the PTS course manual, *Can-Fit-Pro's Foundations of Professional Personal Training,* and the companion study guide. In order to improve your chances of success, we recommend that you attempt the theory exam approximately 3 to 4 weeks after taking the PTS preparatory course. This time frame is designed to help you synthesize the course information while it is still fresh in your mind. Finally, we recommend that you invest approximately 20 hours honing your professional skills before attempting the practical exam. You may attempt the theory and practical exams on the same day, based on the availability of your PRO Trainer for the two examinations.

About Being a Can-Fit-Pro Personal Training Specialist

The Can-Fit-Pro PTS certification meets or exceeds all national standards for certification in Canada. To maintain a consistent standard of excellence from our certified professionals, all must observe the Can-Fit-Pro Certified Fitness Professional Code of Ethics and the scope of ability related to the designations that they hold.

Can-Fit-Pro Certified Fitness Professional Code of Ethics

As a Can-Fit-Pro certified fitness professional, I commit to do the following:

- Educate others to perform safe and effective exercise.
- Motivate others to pursue a healthy, happy, and balanced lifestyle.
- Communicate in a genuine, honest, and professional manner with all individuals.
- Continually strive to learn more about new research and exercise techniques.
- Protect and respect the confidentiality of all my professional fitness relationships at all times.
- Maintain annual CPR training and regular first aid training.
- Respect business, employment, and copyright laws.

- Secure liability insurance to properly protect myself and everyone who is involved with professional fitness services that I provide.
- Work within my scope of ability and refer clients to more qualified professionals in the health care industry when necessary.
- Promote a fit and healthy lifestyle as a positive Can-Fit-Pro role model.

Can-Fit-Pro Personal Training Specialist Scope of Ability

A Can-Fit-Pro–certified PTS is qualified to do the following:

- Evaluate client needs in physical activity and nutrition based on the counseling foundations in the PTS program and provide clients with a safe and effective exercise plan based on their needs, abilities, and goals.
- Confirm that clients have completed the Physical Activity Readiness Questionnaire (PAR-Q), and then provide an individualized training session to apparently healthy individuals who have no known major medical conditions.
- Monitor client resting and exercise heart rate and blood pressure regularly.
- Develop a client-specific exercise plan within clients' level of ability and progress to more advanced training techniques once the proper competency has been achieved.
- Modify all client exercise technique as needed to strive for optimal individual biomechanical effectiveness.
- Promote the benefits of regular physical activity and a balanced lifestyle combined with a healthy diet using Canada's *Physical Activity Guide to Healthy Active Living* as a reference.
- Provide generalized advice on nutrition based on Canada's Food Guide. Clients who require more specific advice on diet and supplements must be referred to a qualified nutrition professional.
- Answer general questions on injuries or discomforts related to exercise. All injuries must be diagnosed and treated by a qualified medical professional.

- Provide emergency care based on participant needs (e.g., contact EMS, provide emergency first aid or CPR).

As a certified PTS, you agree to provide a safe and effective exercise program that provides appropriate exercise selection and intensity to meet the individual needs of each adult client. You agree to respect your role, abide by the code of ethics, and work within your scope of ability at all times. Failure to follow this scope of ability can result in immediate removal of your PTS certification designation.

Importance of Theoretical Concepts and Practical Competencies

To be a personal trainer is to have a solid foundational knowledge of theoretical fitness concepts as well as sound practical competencies to be able to provide safe, effective workouts for clients and provide yourself with the opportunity for a stable income. You must know and be comfortable with the following.

Required Theoretical Concepts

- Benefits of physical activity
- Wellness or holism
- Active living
- Exercise physiology (energy systems, oxygen transport, exercise response)
- Human anatomy (musculoskeletal, cardiorespiratory)
- Biomechanics (joints, levers, modifications, types of contractions)
- Relevance and interpretation of results of fitness assessments
- Principles of conditioning (FITT and SMART)
- Training program design
- Injury prevention and safety
- Basic nutrition (based on Canada's Food Guide)
- Healthy weight management

Required Practical Competencies

- Act ethically and in the best interests of the client at all times.
- Recommend a variety of exercises and training programs for healthy adults.

- Provide safe, effective, and enjoyable workouts.
- Demonstrate strong leadership and communication skills.
- Demonstrate competent administration of a limited number of fitness assessments.
- Demonstrate proper exercise technique.
- Create a client-centred environment.
- Educate clients about how the body responds to exercise.
- Monitor clients' progress and ability.
- Evaluate your training effectiveness.
- Put theoretical knowledge into practice.
- Present a professional appearance.

Practical Exam

To properly prepare for the practical exam, we recommend you practice working through the personal training process, using the following forms to guide you. These are the same forms covered in the course manual, so be sure to refer to the manual when you have questions.

General Written Exam Preparation Guidelines

Special thanks to the University of Windsor and the STEPS program for allowing Can-Fit-Pro to use their information on these pages.

In order to pass the exam, you need to know the material and you also need to be able to demonstrate your knowledge. The testing process can be stressful. In this section, we will outline some procedures that will help make this process a little easier. Your PRO Trainer can always make suggestions beyond what we have listed in this section. As always, don't be shy when asking for help.

General Study Tips

- Be prepared.
- Review regularly.
- Ask for help.
- Carefully listen to tips from your instructor.
- Understand the material rather than simply memorize it.
- Studying effectively means studying actively.
- Work with the information rather than just looking at it.

- Review in groups or with a partner.
- Don't study too long.
- Eat right and get enough sleep.

Before the Exam

- Be informed of when, where, and how long the exam is.
- Be on time.
- Be physically prepared with the following:
  - Calculator
  - Watch
  - Bottle of water
  - Extra pen
- Be mentally focused by eliminating distractions around you.
- Remember that a certain level of pretest anxiety is normal.

What Is Test Anxiety?

- Mental anxiety includes the following:
  - Thoughts and worries about the test
  - Questioning and doubting yourself
- Physical anxiety includes the following:
  - Sensations and tensions
  - Pains and stiffness

Controlling Your Anxiety

- Study effectively.
- Visualize yourself as calm, well prepared, and successful.
- Be confident.
- Practice block breathing: Inhale, count to three, and slowly exhale. Repeat this a few times.
- Practice tensing and relaxing muscles. For example, make a fist and then slowly release it.
- Continue exercising regularly.

During the Exam

- Read the directions carefully.
- Read each question carefully.
- Underline key words.
- Ask for clarification if a question is unclear.
- Preview the entire exam and assess your time constraints and your personal strengths and weaknesses.

- Stick to your time schedule.
- Immediately write down anything you are afraid of forgetting.
- Start with the area you are most confident in.
- Carefully monitor your time.
- Leave yourself enough time to review your answers.

Multiple-Choice Tests

Multiple-choice tests are difficult for several reasons. Answers are worded differently, there are usually many questions, and topic order is altered. In addition, simple recognition is not normally enough. You still need to understand the material and be able to apply your knowledge to various situations.

Preparing for Multiple-Choice Tests

- Begin studying early.
- Identify groups of facts that are similar in meaning.
- Make lists and tables.
- Look for information that can be easily translated into a multiple-choice question.

During the Multiple-Choice Exam

- If you can't answer a question within 1 minute, skip it and come back to it later.
- Look at all the possible answers.
- Underline key words.
- Try answering the question on your own before looking at the possible answers.

Nine Principles of Multiple-Choice Test Taking

1. Choose the answer that the test maker intended. Try not to read into question qualifications and interpretations not intended by the test maker.
2. Anticipate the answer and then look for it.
   - Read the question and then anticipate what facts you think the answer will contain. If the answer you anticipated is found among the options, it's probably correct.
   - Even when you do not know the material, the question will often give clues as to what type of answer the test maker is aiming for.
3. Consider all the alternatives.
   - Read and consider all of the options, even if you find your anticipated answer among the answer choices.

- Because students often jump at the first plausible option, test makers frequently place their most attractive decoy first.
4. Relate the options to the question.
   - When the answer you anticipated is not among the options, discard it and focus on the answers that are there.
   - Systematically consider how each option answers the question.
   - Never deal with answers in isolation. Although the answer may be a true statement, it must still be the correct answer to the question.

Keep in Mind

Even though the answer may be an incorrect statement, it could be the correct answer to the question.

5. Balance options against each other.
   - When several options look good, or if none looks good, compare them with each other.
   - If two options are very similar, study them to find out what makes them different. One of these is likely the correct answer.
   - Look for the answer that is most likely to be correct in comparison with your own anticipated answer and the other choices given.
6. Use logical reasoning.
   - Eliminate those options that you know to be incorrect as well as those that do not fit the requirements of the question.
   - If you recognize more than one of the options as correct, choose the option that best fits the requirements of the question.
7. Look for special cue words.
   - Check the stem of the question for special cue words.
   - Absolute terms, or words that create broad, sweeping generalizations, such as *always, never,* and *without exception,* tend to appear in incorrect statements.
   - Since true statements often have exceptions, they may contain relative terms, such as *sometimes* or *usually,* whereas false ones often do not.

Remember

A statement that includes the word *always* must be true 100% of the time.

A statement that includes the word *never* must also be true 100% of the time.

8. Specific, detailed answers tend to be correct.
   - Although there will be exceptions, options that are more detailed than others tend to be correct.
   - Pay special attention to options that are extra long or highly specific.

9. Use information obtained from other questions and options. Some questions may contain information that may be helpful in answering other questions, especially in tests that cover a small unit of information.

Client Information

Name: _____

Address: _____

Home phone: _____ Work phone: _____

Date of birth:_____ Occupation: _____

Height (cm): _____ Weight (kg): _____

BMI: _____ (BMI = weight in kg / height in m^2)

Systolic BP:_____ mmHg Diastolic BP:_____ mmHg

Pulse: _____ bpm

Please mark each statement that is true.

___ You are a man over the age of 45 years.

___ You are a woman over the age of 55 years.

___ You are physically inactive (active less than 30 minutes, 3 times a week).

___ You are overweight (9 kg or more, or BMI over 30).

___ You presently smoke or have quit within the past 6 months.

___ You have high blood pressure or take blood pressure medication.

   ___ You have systolic blood pressure over 140mmHg.

   ___ You have diastolic blood pressure over 90 mmHg.

___ You have been told you have high cholesterol.

___ Your father or brother had a heart attack or heart surgery before the age of 55.

___ Your mother or sister had a heart attack or heart surgery before the age of 65.

Exercise Habits

___ Intensive occupational and recreational exertion

___ Moderate occupational and recreational exertion

___ Sedentary work and intense recreational exertion

___ Sedentary work and moderate recreational exertion

___ Sedentary work and light recreational exertion

___ Complete lack of occupational or exertion

Is there any reason why you can't exercise regularly? _____

_____

Figure 1 Client health history form.

What exercises do you enjoy or have enjoyed in the past?

1. _____

2. _____

3. _____

Existing Medical Conditions

Please check the appropriate conditions.

___ Anemia   ___ Epilepsy   ___ Thyroid problems

___ Arthritis   ___ Heart condition   ___ Ulcer

___ Asthma   ___ Hernia   ___ Other (please list): _____

___ Cholesterol   ___ Obesity

___ Diabetes   ___ Pregnancy

Medications

Are you currently taking any medications? ___ Yes ___ No

If so, please list the medication and for what condition.

Medication _____ Condition _____

Medication _____ Condition _____

Medication _____ Condition _____

Allergies

Do you have any allergies? ___ Yes ___ No

If so, please list and indicate if medication is required.

Medication _____ Condition _____

Medication _____ Condition _____

Injuries

Do you have pain, or have you injured any of the following areas?

___ Neck   ___ Wrist (R / L)

___ Upper back   ___ Hip (R / L)

___ Lower back   ___ Knee (R / L)

___ Shoulder (R / L)   ___ Ankle (R / L)

___ Elbow (R / L)   Please explain: _____

_____

_____

(continued)

I have seen the following medical practitioners in the past:

	1 month	6 months	12 months
Family physician or other MD	_____	_____	_____
Dentist or orthodontist	_____	_____	_____
Physiotherapis	_____	_____	_____
Chiropractor	_____	_____	_____
Other:_____	_____	_____	_____

Family Physician

Name: _____

City: _____

Phone number: _____

Lifestyle

	Always	Sometimes	Rarely
I get 7-8 hours of sleep per night.	__	__	__
I am physically active 3 times a week.	__	__	__
I have regular medical checkups.	__	__	__
I eat 3-5 servings of vegetables daily.	__	__	__
I eat 2-4 servings of fruit daily.	__	__	__
I eat 6-10 servings of grains and cereals daily.	__	__	__
I eat 2-3 servings of meats and nuts daily.	__	__	__
I make a conscious effort to eat healthy.	__	__	__
I follow a strict diet.	__	__	__
I have no stress in my life.	__	__	__
I am a very happy person.	__	__	__
I am highly motivated.	__	__	__

Comments: _____

_____

_____

Figure 1 *continued*

Client Information

Name: _____ Date: _____

Appraiser: _____

Height (cm): _____

Weight (kg): _____

BMI (kg/m²): _____

Waist girth (cm): _____

Circle the appropriate risk based on BMI and waist girth.

CATEGORY	BMI (KG/M²)	Disease risk relative to normal weight and waist circumference	
		MEN ≤102 CM WOMEN ≤88 CM	MEN >102 CM WOMEN >88 CM
Underweight	≥18.5	—	—
Normal	18.5-24.9	—	—
Overweight	25.0-29.9	Increased	High
Obese I	30.0-34.9	High	Very high
Obese II	35.0-39.9	Very high	Very high
Extremely obese	≥40.0	Extremely high	Extremely high

Bioelectrical Impedance Analysis

Fat-free mass (kg): _____

Fat mass (kg): _____

Goals

1. _____

   _____

2. _____

   _____

Figure 2   Fitness assessment tracking.

Cardiorespiratory Training Plan

Client: _____ Date:_____

Please describe your client's workout.

Counseling

Things to discuss before the workout begins: _____

_____

_____

Warm-Up

Purpose: _____

Intensity (RPE): _____

Duration: _____

Type of activity: _____

Benefits of Cardiorespiratory Training

Purpose: _____

Important points to discuss: _____

_____

Frequency

Number of times a week the client does cardio training:_____

_____

Intensity

HR range (%) of HRmax: _____

HR in BPM (range): _____

RPE (range): _____

Important points to discuss: _____

_____

Time

How long the cardiorespiratory training will last: _____

Important points to discuss: _____

_____

Figure 3 Cardiorespiratory training plan.

Type

What types of equipment the client uses and why: _____

_____

Water

Important points to discuss: _____

_____

Cool-Down

Purpose: _____

Important points to discuss about future workouts: _____

_____

Resistance Training Plan

Client: _____ Date: _____

Please describe your client's workout.

Counseling

Things to discuss before the workout begins: _____

_____

_____

Benefits of Resistance Training

Purpose: _____

Important points to discuss: _____

_____

Frequency

Number of times a week the client does resistance training: _____

_____

Intensity

% 1RM (range): _____

sets to be done: _____

reps (range): _____

Important points to discuss: _____

_____

Time

Rest between sets or exercises: _____

Figure 4 Resistance training plan.

Exercises

Muscles worked and important technique information:

1. _____

2. _____

3. _____

4. _____

5. _____

6. _____

7. _____

8. _____

9. _____

10. _____

11. _____

12. _____

13. _____

14. _____

15. _____

Flexibility Training Plan

Client: _____ Date: _____

Please describe your client's workout.

Benefits of Stretching

Purpose: _____

Important points to discuss: _____

_____

Stretching Technique

Important points to discuss: _____

_____

Exercises

Muscle stretched and important technique points:

1. _____

2. _____

3. _____

4. _____

5. _____

6. _____

7. _____

8. _____

9. _____

10. _____

11. _____

12. _____

13. _____

14. _____

15. _____

Figure 5 Flexibility training plan.

CHAPTER 1

Principles of Fitness, Health, and Wellness Concepts

Mike Bates, MBA
Rod Macdonald, BEd

Multiple-Choice Questions

1. **Which of the following is not one of the primary components of fitness?**
   a. Balance
   b. Body composition
   c. Flexibility
   d. Muscular capacity

2. **Which of the following is not one of the components of performance based fitness?**
   a. Coordination
   b. Agility
   c. Mental capacity
   d. Vertical jump

3. **_____ is the ability to use all body parts together to produce smooth and fluid motion.**
   a. Agility
   b. Speed
   c. Balance
   d. Coordination

4. **_____ is the product of strength and speed.**
   a. Muscular capacity
   b. Power
   c. Cardiorespiratory capacity
   d. Agility

5. **ACSM recommends ____ min or more of moderate-intensity physical activity on most days of the week for cardiovascular health**
   a. 30 min
   b. 10 min
   c. 45 min
   d. 60 min

6. **Which of the following is not one of the recommendations from Canada's Physical Activity Guide to Healthy Active Living**
   a. Flexibility on 4 to 7 days of the week
   b. Strength on 2 to 4 days of the week
   c. Balance training on 2 to 4 days of the week
   d. Endurance activities on 4 to 7 days of the week

7. **This principle suggests that programs and modifications to programs must be made to accommodate every person's individual needs**
   a. FITT
   b. Individualization
   c. Specificity
   d. Progressive overload

8. The following example best demonstrates, which principle: "A client who has a goal of running a marathon should have some exercises included in his program that specifically targets the ankles, knees, hips and back, as these areas will be stressed with marathon training"

   a. Specificity

   b. Individualization

   c. Structural tolerance

   d. FITT

9. This principle suggests that once training ceases, the body will gradually return to a pre-training state

   a. Reversibility

   b. Maintenance

   c. Recovery

   d. Specificity

10. Which of the following is not one of the other components of health that are just as important as physical health?

    a. Social health

    b. Emotional Health

    c. Spiritual Health

    d. Muscular capacity

References

American College of Sports Medicine. 2005 *ACSM's guidelines for exercise testing and prescription,* 7th ed. Philadelphia, PA: Lippincott, Williams and Wilkins.

Brooks, D. 2004. *The complete book of personal training.* Champaign, IL: Human Kinetics. Canadas Physical Activity Guides for Helath: Adults, older adults, children and youth. http://www.phac-aspc.gc.ca/pau-uap/paguide/index.html.

Greenberg, J.S., G.B. Dintiman, and B.M. Oakes. 2004. *Physical fitness and wellness,* 3rd ed. Champaign, IL: Human Kinetics.

Zaryski, C., and Smith, D.J. 2005. Training principles and issues for ultra-endurance athletes. *Current Sports Medicine Reports* 4: 165-170.

CHAPTER 2

Nutrition Concepts for Personal Trainers

Brian Justin, MHK

Gregory S. Anderson, PhD

Key Terms

nutrition

essential nutrient

glycemic index

vitamins

minerals

ergogenic aids

Canada's Food Guide

Review Questions

1. What are the six essential nutrients and their function in maintaining health?

   _____

   _____

   _____

   _____

   _____

   _____

2. What is the difference between a simple carbohydrate and a complex carbohydrate?

   _____

   _____

3. Carbohydrate provides fuel for _____and _____, and it provides fibre for_____
   _____.

4. _____ represent 95% of all fat we eat.

5. Carbohydrate has _____ calories per gram, whereas every gram of fat provides _____ calories.

6. The major role of _____ is to build and repair the tissues of the body.

7. What percentage of total daily calories should be consumed as each of the following?
   a. carbohydrate _____
   b. fat _____
   c. protein _____

8. What are the two groups of vitamins?

   _____

   _____

9. About _____% of human body mass is water.

10. What five strategies can you use to move your clients toward healthy eating?

    _____

    _____

    _____

    _____

    _____

Multiple-Choice Questions

1. **Personal trainers are certified to provide**
   a. diet analysis
   b. diet modification
   c. ergogenic supplementation prescriptions
   d. general nutrition advice

2. **Which of the following is *not* a macronutrient?**
   a. carbohydrate
   b. vitamin A
   c. protein
   d. fat

3. **Which of the following is a simple carbohydrate?**
   a. bread
   b. pasta
   c. honey
   d. vegetables

4. **The average Canadian drinks how many litres of pop a year?**
   a. 50
   b. 40
   c. 100
   d. 200

5. **What is the required intake of fibre for women?**
   a. 25 grams
   b. 38 grams
   c. 32 grams
   d. 20 grams

6. **The higher the intensity of exercise, the greater reliance on**
   a. protein
   b. fat
   c. carbohydrate
   d. water

7. **Carbohydrate yields how many calories per gram?**
   a. 5
   b. 4
   c. 9
   d. 7

8. **Which type of fat represents 95% of the fat we consume?**
   a. sterols
   b. phospholipids
   c. wax
   d. triglycerides

9. **Fat yields how many calories per gram?**
   a. 9
   b. 7
   c. 8
   d. 10

10. **Which fat source should *not* be included in a healthy diet?**
    a. avocado
    b. salmon
    c. hydrogenated palm oil
    d. almonds

11. **Which of the following is *not* a function of fat?**
    a. hormone production
    b. energy
    c. source of vitamin B
    d. taste enhancement

12. **Which of the following is *not* a function of protein?**
    a. primary source of energy
    b. muscle tissue building
    c. hormone production
    d. enzyme creation

13. **Which recommendation will *not* maximize your dietary vitamin intake?**
    a. Eat a variety of colourful fruits and vegetables.
    b. Eat fresh fruits and vegetables as much as possible, especially those in season.
    c. Eat a variety of processed foods.
    d. Don't overcook vegetables; keep them a little crunchy.

14. **Which of the following functions does iodine perform?**
    a. regulates body fluid levels
    b. essential in bone health
    c. important in the formation of hemoglobin
    d. regulates metabolism

15. **Which of the following is not a function of water?**
    a. digestion and metabolism
    b. assisting with chemical reactions
    c. lubricating joints
    d. none of the above

References

Armstrong, L. 2000. *Performing in extreme environments*. Champaign, IL: Human Kinetics.

Benardot, D. 2006. *Advanced sports nutrition*. Champaign, IL: Human Kinetics.

Brooks, D. 2004. *The complete book of personal training*. Champaign, IL: Human Kinetics.

Canada's Guide to Healthy Eating and Physical Activity. http://www.phac-aspc.gc.ca/guide/index_e.html.

Centre for Nutrition Policy and Promotion. My Pyramid. http://www.cnpp.usda.gov/

Enig, M. 2000. *Know your fats: The complete primer for understanding the nutrition of fats, oils, and cholesterol*. Silver Spring, MD: Bethesda Press.

Thompson, J., M. Manore, and J. Sheeshka. 2007. *Nutrition: A functional approach*, Canadian Edition. Toronto, Ontario: Pearson Education Canada.

CHAPTER 3

Bioenergetics Concepts

Brian Justin, MHK

Gregory S. Anderson, PhD

Key Terms

- bioenergetics
- energy
- metabolism
- adenosine triphosphate (ATP)
- creatine phosphate (CP)
- anaerobic threshold
- anaerobic glycolysis
- aerobic system
- work-to-rest ratio
- energy continuum

Review Questions

1. **What is ATP?**

   _____

2. **Name the three energy systems, and indicate if they require oxygen or if lactic acid is produced.**

   _____

   _____

   _____

3. **How long will the ATP–CP system sustain activity?**

   _____

4. **The glycolytic system breaks down _____ and produces _____.**

5. **The only energy pathway that can burn carbohydrate, fat, and protein is the _____**

   _____.

6. **Describe the energy production that occurs as you move from rest to moderate-intensity exercise.**

   _____

7. **What is the importance of the anaerobic threshold to a marathon runner?**

   _____

8. **What is excess post-exercise oxygen consumption (EPOC), and why does it occur?**

   _____

9. **Fill in the chart concerning the energy systems.**

SYSTEM	RATE AND AMOUNT OF ATP PRODUCTION	FUEL USED	CAPACITY OF SYSTEM	MAJOR LIMITATION	PRIMARY USE
ATP–CP (anaerobic)			Very limited		
Glycolytic (anaerobic)				Lactic acid by-product (causes fatigue)	
CHO oxidation (aerobic)	Slow rate (38 ATP/unit of glucose)				
Fatty acid oxidation (aerobic)		Fatty acids in bloodstream			Low intensity and 2+ minutes

10. **Describe the proper work-to-rest intervals for developing the ATP–CP system and the required work intensity.**

_____

11. **Provide examples of sports or activities that use each energy system as their predominant energy pathway.**

ATP–CP system: _____

Anaerobic glycolysis: _____

Aerobic system: _____

Multiple-Choice Questions

1. **The energy currency of the body is**
   a. carbohydrate
   b. fat
   c. ATP
   d. ADP

2. **The ATP–CP system can fuel activity for approximately how many seconds?**
   a. 30
   b. 10
   c. 28.5
   d. 3

3. **The glycolytic energy pathway consists of how many enzymatically driven reactions?**
   a. 10
   b. 15
   c. 12
   d. 8

4. **Glycolysis will produce energy for movement up to**
   a. 4 minutes
   b. 60 seconds
   c. 120 seconds
   d. 1 minute

5. **The final by-products of aerobic metabolism are**
   a. carbon dioxide and water
   b. carbonic acid
   c. pyruvic acid
   d. urea

6. **Fatty acid oxidation results in the production of how many ATP molecules?**
   a. 25
   b. 38
   c. 100
   d. 120

7. **If you have to sprint to a bus that is 40 metres away, what energy system will predominate for energy production?**

   a. Glycolytic system

   b. ATP–CP system

   c. Aerobic metabolism

   d. Oxidative pathway

8. **Which statement best describes the anaerobic threshold?**

   a. the point at which a person begins to feel nauseated

   b. the point at which the aerobic system cannot supply enough ATP for the needs of the body

   c. the point at which a person transitions from rest to movement

   d. the point at which a person transitions from walking to running

9. **EPOC serves which of the following functions?**

   a. ATP and CP replenishment

   b. resolution of the disequilibrium in physiologic functions

   c. reloading of oxygen to the myoglobin in muscles

   d. all of the above

10. **Which energy system is best for rapidly producing ATP?**

    a. lactic acid system

    b. aerobic system

    c. ATP-CP system

    d. b and c

11. **What is produced in the muscles when effort exceeds the oxygen supply?**

    a. amino acids

    b. lactic acid

    c. creatine phosphate

    d. PFK

12. **High-intensity interval conditioning is appropriate for which population?**

    a. sedentary people

    b. beginning exercisers

    c. elite athletes

    d. bowlers

13. **What type of relief should you use between work bouts in order to develop the ATP–CP system?**

    a. rest

    b. work

    c. skipping

    d. jogging

14. A person running a standard marathon relies predominately on what system?

    a. ATP–CP

    b. glycolytic system

    c. aerobic system

    d. a and b

15. Which statement is correct regarding the energy systems?

    a. At any time all of the energy systems are being used and system predominance depends on intensity and duration.

    b. Heavy weight training helps develop the aerobic system.

    c. Golf mainly uses the oxidative system.

    d. Conditioning the anaerobic system daily is essential for development.

References

Brooks, D. 2004. *The complete book of personal training.* Champaign, IL: Human Kinetics.

Griffin, J. 2006. *Client-centered exercise prescription,* 2nd ed. Champaign, IL: Human Kinetics.

Hoffman, J. 2002. *Physiological aspects of sport training and performance.* Champaign, IL: Human Kinetics.

McArdle, W., F. Katch, and V. Katch. 2007. *Exercise physiology: Energy, nutrition, and human performance,* 6th ed. Baltimore, MD: Lippincott, Williams and Wilkins.

National Strength and Conditioning Association. 2000. *Essentials of strength training and conditioning,* 2nd ed. Champaign, IL: Human Kinetics.

National Strength and Conditioning Association: Performance Training Journal. http://www.nsca-lift.org/Perform/backissues.asp.

Sharkey, B., and S. Gaskill. 2006. *Sport physiology for coaches.* Champaign, IL: Human Kinetics.

Siff, M. 2003. *Supertraining.* Denver, CO: Supertraining Institute.

Twist Conditioning Inc. 2004. *Sport movement specialist certification course handouts.* North Vancouver, BC: Twist Conditioning Inc.

Whyte, G. 2006. *Physiology of training.* London, UK: Churchill Livingstone Elsevier.

CHAPTER 4

Cardiorespiratory Concepts

Gregory S. Anderson, PhD
Brian Justin, MHK

Key Terms

- pulmonary circulation
- systemic circulation
- atria
- ventricle
- blood pressure (BP)
- cardiac output
- ventilation
- $\dot{V}O_2max$
- central training effects
- peripheral training effects
- target heart rate (HR)

Review Questions

1. Define *artery* and *vein*.

   _____

   _____

2. The _____ pushes blood to the body tissues, including the muscles.

3. The right side of the heart receives blood from _____ and moves it into _____ _____ circulation.

4. Blood leaves the heart in vessels referred to as _____.

5. At rest, the average adult pumps _____ litres of blood per minute.

6. During exercise, _____ BP rises rapidly, while _____ BP remains fairly constant.

7. Why can HR be used to predict exercise intensity?

   _____

   _____

8. Write an equation that defines cardiac output.

   _____

9. A fit person and an unfit person both pump the same amount of blood at rest. The fit person has a _____ HR because the stroke volume is _____.

10. What tissues have the greatest change in blood flow during exercise?

    _____

    _____

11. What is $\dot{V}O_2$max? Why is it important to endurance athletes?

    _____

    _____

12. List three central and three peripheral training effects that occur as a result of aerobic training.

    _____

    _____

    _____

    _____

    _____

    _____

13. **Use two different methods to calculate the target HR zone for a 50-year-old female who has a resting HR of 80 beats per minute (bpm) and a low fitness level.**

    a. percentage maximum heart rate (HRmax): _____

    b. heart rate reserve (HRR): _____

14. **A rating of perceived exertion (RPE) of 12 on a 20-point scale would be classified using a verbal descriptor as _____; the percentage of HRmax related to this intensity would be between _____% and _____ %.**

15. **List the optimal recommendation for each of the following.**

    a. frequency of training: _____

    b. duration of training: _____

    c. intensity of training: _____

16. **Define the FITT formula and offer suggestions regarding each aspect for someone of average fitness.**

_____

_____

Anatomical Structures

Label the indicated parts in the anatomical structures that follow.

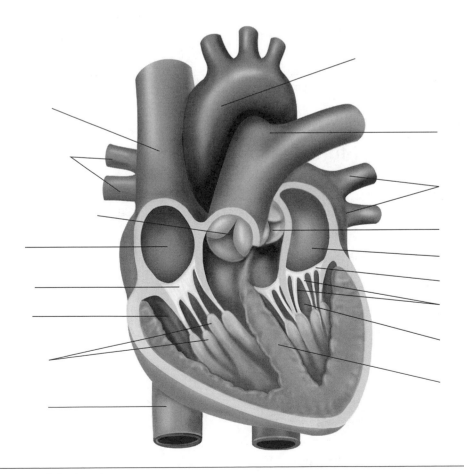

Figure 6   Anatomy of the heart.

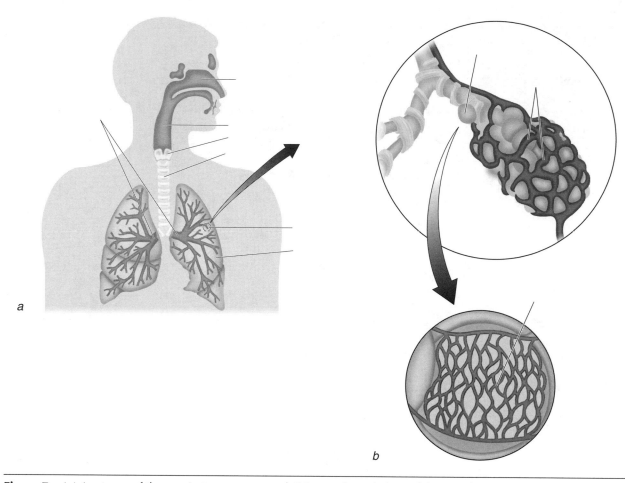

Figure 7   *(a)* Anatomy of the respiratory system and *(b)* an enlarged view of the aveolus.

Multiple-Choice Questions

1. **Your V̇O₂ max is**
   a. indicative of your maximum aerobic energy yields
   b. the greatest amount of oxygen you can extract and utilize per unit of time
   c. a measure of your aerobic capacity
   d. all of the above

2. **You can increase cardiac output during exercise by**
   a. increasing stroke volume
   b. decreasing resting HR
   c. increasing BP
   d. all of the above

3. **The respiratory system is responsible for**
   a. gas exchange between the lungs and blood
   b. moving air into and out of the lungs
   c. removing carbon dioxide from the blood
   d. all of the above

4. **Systolic BP is**
   a. the peak pressure developed during the ejection phase
   b. the lowest pressure developed during the filling phase
   c. the result of hypertension
   d. the amount of blood pumped from the heart with each heartbeat

5. **The target HR range for a healthy 20-year-old male should be**
   a. 110 to 150 bpm
   b. 120 to 170 bpm
   c. 140 to 190 bpm
   d. 110 to 180 bpm

6. **The Borg scale for prescribing exercise intensity is based on**
   a. the lactate threshold
   b. a percentage of $\dot{V}O_2$max
   c. a percentage of HRmax
   d. perceived exertion

7. **Cooling down after activity prevents**
   a. venous blood pooling
   b. delayed muscle soreness
   c. fatigue
   d. heart disease

8. **For program design, consider**
   a. the client's exercise experience
   b. the client's current fitness and activity level
   c. the client's goals for cardiorespiratory conditioning
   d. all of the above

9. **An exercise intensity described as *somewhat hard* is equivalent to**
   a. an RPE of 14 to 16
   b. an HR between 65% and 80% of HRR
   c. an HR of 60% to 79% of HRmax
   d. all of the above

10. **A 40-year-old female with a resting HR of 75 bpm would have a minimum HR of ____ to be in the target HR zone using the HRR method.**
    a. 122 bpm
    b. 128 bpm
    c. 142 bpm
    d. 135 bpm

11. **Which of the following increases $\dot{V}O_2$max by increasing oxygen extraction?**
    a. increased capillary density
    b. increased stroke volume
    c. increased BP
    d. increased red blood cells

12. The air we breathe in is

a. 100% oxygen

b. 65% oxygen

c. 34% oxygen

d. 21% oxygen

13. At rest, the muscles receive _____ % of the total blood moved from the heart, whereas during exercise this can be _____ %.

a. 4; 100

b. 20; 84

c. 27; 75

d. 21; 58

14. Untrained people will have a higher resting HR because they

a. require more oxygen at rest

b. have high BP

c. have a lower stroke volume

d. all of the above

References

Canada's Physical Activity Guides for Health: Adults, older adults, children and youth. http://www.phac-aspc.gc.ca/pau-uap/paguide/index.html.

Centres for Disease Control and Prevention. Physical Activity for Everyone. http://www.cdc.gov/nccdphp/dnpa/physical/index.htm.

McArdle, W., F. Katch, and V. Katch. 2007. *Exercise physiology: Energy, nutrition, and human performance*, 6th ed. Baltimore, MD: Lippincott, Williams and Wilkins.

National Strength and Conditioning Association: Performance Training Journal. http://www.nsca-lift.org/Perform/backissues.asp.

CHAPTER 5

Skeletal Anatomy and Flexibility Concepts

Carmen Bott, MSc

Key Terms

- axial skeleton
- appendicular skeleton
- joints
- synovial joints
- flexibility
- static stretching
- dynamic stretching

Review Questions

1. **List four functions of the skeletal system.**

   _____

   _____

   _____

   _____

2. **There are _____ bones in the body, of which most are found in the _____ _____ skeleton.**

3. **List the four classifications of bones and give an example of each classification.**

   _____

   _____

   _____

   _____

4. **List the three classifications of joints and give an example of each classification.**

   _____

   _____

   _____

5. **Identify the anatomical names for the following bones:**

   shoulder blade: _____

   forearm: _____

   shinbone: _____

   kneecap: _____

   collar bone: _____

   thigh bone: _____

6. **Following are some common joints in the body. Identify the type of joint and what bones articulate to form it.**

   hip: _____

   knee: _____

   shoulder: _____

   elbow: _____

   wrist: _____

   ankle: _____

7. **What is the difference between the axial and the appendicular skeletons?**

    _____

8. **Define the following anatomical reference terms, and provide the term that is used to identify the opposite.**

    anterior: _____

    medial: _____

    inferior: _____

    supine: _____

    prone: _____

    distal: _____

    flexion: _____

    abduction: _____

9. **List the four major benefits of flexibility training.**

    _____

    _____

    _____

    _____

10. **Explain the difference between static and dynamic stretching.**

    _____

11. **List ways in which you could modify a stretch.**

    _____

    _____

Anatomical Structures

Label the indicated parts in the following illustrations.

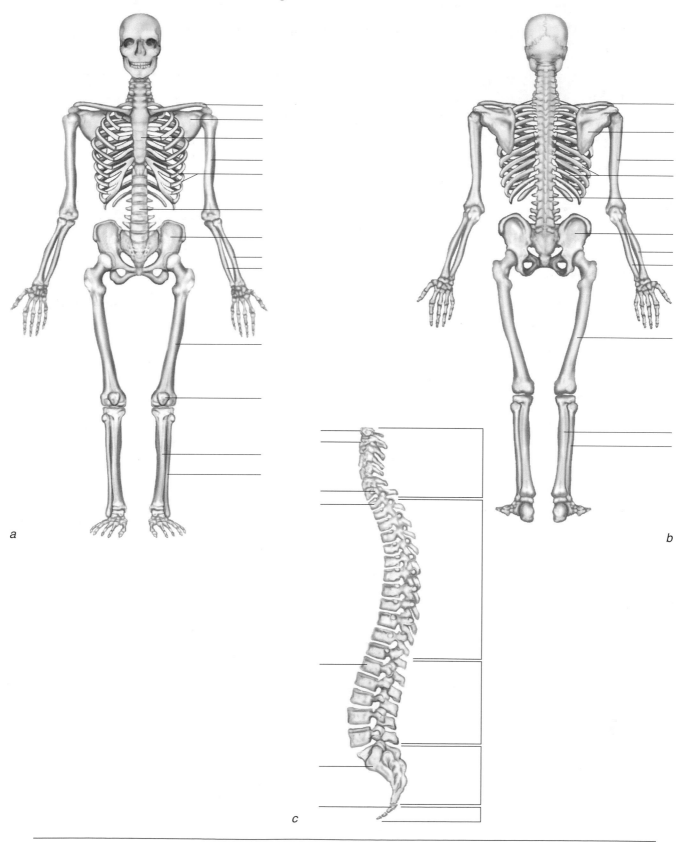

Figure 8 Anatomy of the *(a)* anterior and *(b)* posterior skeleton and *(c)* of the vertebral column.

Multiple-Choice Questions

1. **The skeleton provides all of the following essential functions** *except*
   a. protects the vital organs and soft tissue
   b. is the factory where red blood cells are produced
   c. acts a reservoir for minerals (calcium and phosphate)
   d. provides attachments for organs and blood vessels

2. **What are the three categories of joints?**
   a. fibrous, cartilaginous, and synovial
   b. fibrous, synovial, and arthritic
   c. cartilaginous, fibrous, and syndesmoses
   d. cartilaginous, synovial, and fixed

3. **A lever system consists of all of the following** *except*
   a. a bone to act as the lever
   b. a joint that is the fulcrum or axis of rotation
   c. muscular force applied to the lever that causes motion
   d. two muscle groups and a fixed joint angle

4. **In extension, the joint angle becomes**
   a. larger
   b. smaller
   c. weaker
   d. stronger

5. **Which type of vertebrae is the largest?**
   a. thoracic
   b. sacral
   c. lumbar
   d. cervical

6. **The longest bone in the body is the**
   a. tibia
   b. ulna
   c. patella
   d. femur

References

Fu, F., and S. Lephart. 2000. *Proprioception and neuromuscular control in joint stability.* Champaign, IL: Human Kinetics.

National Strength and Conditioning Association. 2000. *Essentials of strength training and conditioning,* 2nd ed. Champaign, IL: Human Kinetics.

Siff, M. 2003. *Supertraining.* Denver, CO: Supertraining Institute.

CHAPTER 6

Muscular Concepts

Carmen Bott, MSc

Key Terms

- muscle fibre
- sarcomere
- concentric contraction
- eccentric contraction
- peripheral nervous system (PNS)
- proprioceptors
- motor unit
- fast-twitch muscle fibre
- slow-twitch muscle fibre
- prime mover
- antagonist
- muscular strength
- muscular power
- muscular endurance
- superset
- split training

Review Questions

1. The smallest functional unit of a muscle is the _____.

2. The two proteins that create tension in the muscle (allow contraction) are _____ and _____.

3. What is the difference between an eccentric and concentric contraction? Use the biceps muscle as an example in your explanation.

   _____

4. When a muscle contracts against large forces and there is no movement or change in muscle length, it is referred to as a _____ contraction.

5. Fill in the following chart.

	SLOW TWITCH	FAST TWITCH
Contraction speed		
Force produced		
Rate of fatigue		
Energy system		

6. **List the six factors related to muscular strength.**

   _____

   _____

   _____

   _____

   _____

   _____

7. **If the following muscles are acting as the prime mover (agonist), what muscles act as the antagonist?**

   quadriceps: _____

   triceps: _____

   rectus abdominis: _____

   gastrocnemius: _____

   trapezius: _____

8. **Provide the primary functions of the following muscles, and list two exercises that can be used to develop each.**

MUSCLE	FUNCTION	EXERCISES TO DEVELOP MUSCLE
Biceps		1. 2.
Deltoid		1. 2.
Pectoralis major		1. 2.
Rectus abdominis		1. 2.
Latissimus dorsi		1. 2.
Erector spinae		1. 2.
Gluteus maximus		1. 2.
Hamstrings		1. 2.
Quadriceps		1. 2.
Gastrocnemius		1. 2.
Tibialis anterior		1. 2.

9. **List ways that resistance training benefits clients.**

    _____
    _____
    _____

10. **What are the eight principles of program design for resistance training?**

    _____
    _____
    _____
    _____
    _____
    _____
    _____
    _____
    _____

11. **Setting the intensity of resistance training includes consideration of three factors: _____, _____, and _____.**

12. **What are supersets and why would you use them?**

    _____

13. **What is split training and why would you use that style of training?**

    _____

14. **List spotting guidelines for both upper- and lower-body exercises.**

    _____

15. **In the following chart, which muscles are involved in the listed exercises?**

EXERCISE	JOINTS	MOVEMENTS	MUSCLE
Squat	Hip Knee Ankle	Extension Extension Plantar flexion	- - -
Toe raise	Ankle	Dorsiflexion	-
Arm curl	Elbow	Flexion	-
Lat pull-down	Shoulder Elbow	Extension Flexion	- -
Bench press	Shoulder Elbow	Horizontal adduction Extension	- -

16. In the following chart, which actions are performed by the listed muscles?

JOINT	MOVEMENT	MUSCLES
Scapula	-	Trapezius (upper)
Shoulder	-	Latissimus dorsi
Elbow	-	Biceps brachii
Spinal	-	Rectus abdominis
Spinal	-	Internal and external obliques
Hip	-	Gluteus medius
Hip	-	Gluteus maximus and hamstrings
Knee	-	Quadriceps
Ankle	-	Gastrocnemius and soleus
Ankle	-	Tibialis anterior

17. In the following chart, which muscles are used at the listed joint during a chin-up?

CHIN-UP	JOINT	MUSCLE
Up phase	Shoulder	-
	Elbow	-
Down phase	Shoulder	-
	Elbow	-

Anatomical Structures

Label the indicated parts in the anatomical structures that follow.

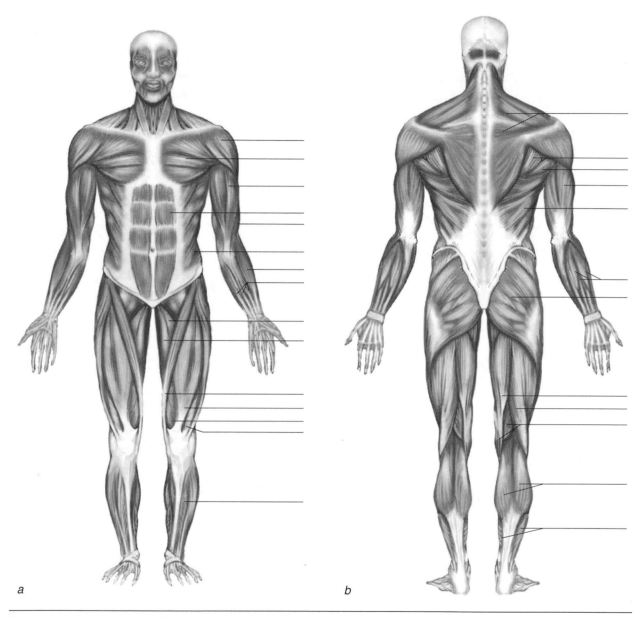

a

b

Figure 9   *(a)* Anterior and *(b)* posterior views of skeletal musculature.

Multiple-Choice Questions

1. **Muscles are attached to bones by**
   a. ligaments
   b. tendons
   c. synergists
   d. prime movers

2. **The prime mover for elbow extension is the**
   a. biceps
   b. triceps
   c. deltoid
   d. pectoralis minor

3. **The basic unit of muscle contraction is**
   a. the myofibril
   b. the muscle fibre
   c. the sarcomere
   d. actin

4. **The main responsibility of the PNS is to**
   a. deliver information about all body parts to the brain for processing
   b. deliver information from the brain to the activated muscles
   c. receive information from the muscles to produce coordinated movement
   d. none of the above

5. **The golgi tendon organ (GTO) is active when**
   a. the muscle spindles send a signal
   b. the tendon contracts
   c. the muscle is relaxed
   d. the tendon is relaxed

6. **Muscle balance as it relates to a resistance training program means**
   a. there should be equal focus on both the antagonist and the agonist muscle groups
   b. equal weight is lifted on all muscle groups
   c. the upper body and lower body should be trained on separate days
   d. none of the above

7. **The FITT formula stands for**
   a. frequency, intensity, type, and training
   b. fast-twitch, intensity, type, and time
   c. frequency, intensity, type, and time
   d. frequency, intensity, total load, and time

8. **In the first 6 to 8 weeks of a resistance training program, beginners experience significant results. This is due to**
   a. improvements in technique
   b. improvements in motor unit recruitment
   c. improved cardiorespiratory performance
   d. good spotting techniques

9. **When the muscle length does not change, the action is**
   a. isotonic
   b. concentric
   c. eccentric
   d. isometric

10. **The benefits of regular resistance training include all of the following** *except*

   a. increases in muscle fibre size
   b. increases in contractile strength
   c. increases in bone and ligament strength
   d. increases in flexibility

11. **The recommended repetition range for a beginner is**

   a. 12 to 15
   b. 15 to 20
   c. 8 to 10
   d. fewer than 8

References

ACSM Brochures: http://www.acsm.org/AM/Template.cfm?Section=Brochures2

Brooks, D. 2004. *The complete book of personal training.* Champaign, IL: Human Kinetics.

McArdle, W., F. Katch, and V. Katch. 2007. *Exercise physiology: Energy, nutrition, and human performance,* 6th ed. Baltimore, MD: Lippincott, Williams and Wilkins.

National Strength and Conditioning Association. 2000. *Essentials of strength training and conditioning,* 2nd ed. Champaign, IL: Human Kinetics.

National Strength and Conditioning Association: Performance Training Journal. http://www.nsca-lift.org/Perform/backissues.asp.

CHAPTER 7

Injury Recognition

Terry Kane, BPHE, BSc

Key Terms

scope of practice

acute injury

overuse injury

sprain

strain

sign

symptom

rest, ice, compression, and elevation

intrinsic risk factor

extrinsic risk factor

Review Questions

1. Differentiate between mechanical and systemic pain.

   _____

   _____

2. Define *scope of practice*. How does it relate to a personal trainer working with an injured client?

   _____

   _____

3. What type of injury is the result of repetitive loading resulting in the gradual onset of pain?

   _____

4. When excessive forces are applied to bones, the bones _____, whereas ligaments _____ _____ and muscles _____.

5. A _____ of an injury is something you can see or measure, whereas a _____ _____ is something the client feels.

6. True or false: For liability protection, you should discontinue exercising with injured clients until they tell you they feel better and want to continue.

   _____

7. Risks of injury related to the exercise environment are considered _____ risk factors.

8. Describe the signs and symptoms of an overuse injury. (Put them in separate lists.)

   _____

   _____

9. As a personal trainer, what are your responsibilities in regard to injury prevention?

   _____

   _____

Multiple-Choice Questions

1. **Which of the following statements is incorrect?**
   a. Pain is how the body tells us that something is wrong and needs investigation and possible treatment or repair.
   b. If ignored or mismanaged, pain can result in permanent disability and even death.
   c. Mechanical pain is the result of damage to the musculoskeletal system in which pain is created by a mechanical action or motion
   d. Systemic pain is not the result of a mechanical action but rather the result of a disease, infection, or medical condition.
   e. None of the above is incorrect.

2. **Which of the following statements is incorrect?**

   a. *Scope of practice* refers to the actions for which a person has been educated and considered competent, usually following successful completion of an examination by a recognized professional or academic organization.

   b. Depending on their knowledge of anatomy and experience, diagnosing a client's pain is within the scope of practice of some personal trainers.

   c. Until given medical clearance from a physician, clients with undiagnosed pain should be instructed to discontinue exercising the injured body region.

   d. None of the above is incorrect.

3. **Which of the following statements is incorrect?**

   a. There are two categories of musculoskeletal injury, defined by their mechanism of injury and onset of symptoms.

   b. An acute injury typically results from the rapid application of a single force or load, resulting in immediate pain and dysfunction.

   c. An overuse injury typically results from repetitive loading, resulting in the gradual onset of pain and dysfunction over days or weeks.

   d. None of the above is incorrect.

4. **Which of the following statements is incorrect?**

   a. A client's age, genetics, history of prior injury, and tissue fatigue can raise or lower the threshold of tissue strength and change the risk of acute injury.

   b. It is important to conduct an initial interview and screening assessment of your client to identify potential problems before designing an exercise program.

   c. Due to the differences in the tensile strength of one tissue to another, from one person to another, and from one activity to another, it is common practice for personal trainers to individualize exercise programs to prevent injury.

   d. None of the above is incorrect.

5. **Which of the following statements is incorrect?**

   a. Clients will typically describe their injury based on how the injury feels and the resulting impact of the injury.

   b. Signs of an acute injury can include immediate swelling at the site of injury, bruising, redness and increased warmth at the site of injury, tenderness to touch, loss of normal function at the site of injury, loss of muscle strength, or loss of motion.

   c. Symptoms of an acute injury can include immediate swelling at the site of injury, bruising, redness and increased warmth at the site of injury, tenderness to touch, loss of normal function at the site of injury, loss of muscle strength, or loss of motion.

   d. None of the above is incorrect.

6. **Which of the following statements is incorrect?**

   a. The goals in the immediate management of an acute injury are minimizing the tissue damage at the injury site and minimizing the inflammatory response associated with the injury.

   b. If excessive inflammation establishes itself at the site of injury, it can increase treatment time and delay a return to activity.

   c. Once the pain has disappeared in an overuse injury, clients can return immediately to their preinjury exercise program without modifying the dose of exercise.

   d. None of the above is incorrect.

7. **Which of the following statements is not an example of an acute injury?**
   a. carpal tunnel syndrome
   b. ligament sprain
   c. muscle strain
   d. fractured bone
   e. Achilles tendon rupture

8. **Which of the following statements is incorrect?**
   a. Any client with acute undiagnosed pain should be referred to a physician for a diagnosis as soon as possible.
   b. Rest facilitates the formation of a primitive scar at the site of injury and varies depending on the injured tissue.
   c. Heat reduces muscle spasm, reduces the immediate inflammatory response, and reduces swelling at the site of injury.
   d. None of the above is incorrect.

9. **Which of the following statements is incorrect?**
   a. Your first recommendation to any injured client with undiagnosed pain should be to see a physician.
   b. For liability protection, you should discontinue exercising with any injured client until such time as you receive written endorsement from a physician that it is safe to continue.
   c. Clients who are currently undergoing treatment for an injury should contact the treating health care professional to determine if exercising with you is indicated or contraindicated at that time.
   d. None of the above is incorrect.

10. **Which of the following statements is incorrect?**
    a. Intrinsic risk factors are personal to the client, such as muscle weakness, muscle inflexibility, muscle imbalances, joint laxity, discrepancy in leg length, degenerative changes, history of surgery, and psychological state of mind and cognitive function.
    b. Extrinsic risk factors are external or environmental factors and include the personal training studio, equipment, and fitness apparel and running shoes worn by your client.
    c. Personal trainers have a responsibility to prevent injuries by screening clients for intrinsic risk factors and minimizing external risk factors.
    d. None of the above is incorrect.

11. **As a personal trainer, it's your responsibility to prevent acute injuries by**
    a. using the client profile to select the safest and most appropriate exercises for your client
    b. using the client profile to determine the best dose (frequency, intensity, volume) of exercise for your client
    c. ensuring that your client is instructed on proper exercise technique in all exercises, including warming up and cooling down
    d. ensuring that your client can independently demonstrate safe execution of all exercises, including safe operation of any associated exercise equipment
    e. all of the above

12. **In terms of overuse injuries, which of the following statements is correct?**
    a. If a given exercise is repeated without adequate time to recover and repair, there can be an accumulation of tissue damage and inflammation.
    b. Tendinitis, shoulder impingement, and patellofemoral pain are examples of common overuse injuries.
    c. To prevent reinjury, clients with a history of recent overuse injury may need to modify their exercise program for 6 months or longer.
    d. All of the above are correct.

13. **Which of the following statements is incorrect?**
    a. Symptoms of an overuse injury can include discomfort in daily activities such as descending stairs or walking.
    b. Signs of an overuse injury can include an alteration of normal biomechanics, swelling, loss of pain-free motion, and tenderness to touch.
    c. The low level of pain and gradual onset associated with overuse injuries often mislead clients into believing their pain is insignificant, that it will go away by itself, and that it does not require medical attention.
    d. None of the above is incorrect.

14. **Which of the following statements is correct?**
    a. Continuing to exercise or do any activity that reproduces pain will only make an injury worse and can result in permanent disability.
    b. Safely returning to exercise after an overuse injury is not necessarily about training hard, but rather about training smart.
    c. Prevention strategies in overuse injuries focuses on three concepts: educating the client, modifying the dose and volume of exercise, and progressing the exercise program slowly.
    d. All of the above are correct.

15. **Which of the following statements is incorrect?**
    a. For all intents and purposes, overuse injuries are unpreventable.
    b. The concept of stopping exercise is difficult for clients who believe in the old saying, "No pain, no gain."
    c. Clients often don't mention their pain until it's too late and they require medical treatment and time off in order to heal.
    d. None of the above is incorrect.

16. **As a personal trainer, it's your responsibility is to prevent overuse injuries by**
    a. educating clients that exercising a painful muscle or joint will only make their pain worse and potentially force them to discontinue exercise
    b. creating an environment where clients feel comfortable telling you that they are sore without fear of ridicule or embarrassment
    c. asking your clients before every training session if they are pain free
    d. modifying or discontinuing any exercise known to cause your client pain
    e. all of the above

CHAPTER 8

Preexercise Screening

Gregory S. Anderson, PhD
Brian Justin, MHK

Key Terms

duty of care

known disease

signs and symptoms

cardiac risk

health risk stratification

Review Questions

1. **List five things that prescreening allows a personal trainer to do.**

    _____

    _____

    _____

    _____

    _____

2. **List the cardiac risks factors that you should screen for as a personal trainer.**

    _____

    _____

3. **Men over the age of _____ years and women over the age of _____ years are encouraged to have a medical exam before initiating an exercise program.**

4. **The Physical Activity Readiness Questionnaire (PAR-Q) is a screening tool that helps assess topics in both the _____ and _____ categories.**

5. **Clients who answer _____ to one or more questions on the PAR-Q should seek medical advice before becoming more physically active.**

6. **Describe a client who is at increased risk and what type of program could be safely started under close supervision.**

    _____

    _____

Multiple-Choice Questions

1. **Negligence may occur when**
    a. there is a breach of the duty to exercise due care
    b. someone gets injured
    c. someone dies
    d. you do not fill your client's expectations

2. **Which of the following is *not* a cardiac risk factor?**
    a. smoking
    b. high BP
    c. being a male over 35 years old
    d. sedentary lifestyle

3. **Preexercise screening must be able to identify those individuals who have any of the following:**

 a. risks inherent in activity due to their age

 b. signs and symptoms of a disease that is as of yet undiagnosed

 c. increased cardiac risk

 d. all of the above

4. **The PAR-Q**

 a. is a waiver for people between 15 and 75 years old

 b. identifies cardiac risk factors

 c. provides informed consent for physical activity

 d. identifies people who should seek medical advice before becoming more physically active

5. **An apparently healthy individual is one who**

 a. answered *yes* to all questions on the PAR-Q

 b. has no more than three cardiac risk factors

 c. can start a moderate-intensity exercise program without a medical referral

 d. exhibits no more than two signs and symptoms of disease

References

ACSM Brochures: Pre-participation Physical Examinations: http://www.acsm.org/Content/ContentFolders/Publications/Brochures/prepart022702.pdf.

American College of Sports Medicine. 2003. *ACSM's exercise management for persons with chronic diseases and disabilities,* 2nd ed. Champaign, IL: Human Kinetics.

CSEP: PAR-Q, PARmedX: http://www.csep.ca/forms.asp.

Delforge, G. 2002. *Musculoskeletal trauma – Implications for sports injury management.* Champaign, IL: Human Kinetics.

Health Screen (Release 1.0). Human Kinetics Software. Champaign, IL: Human Kinetics.

Houglum, P. 2005. *Therapeutic exercise for musculoskeletal injuries,* 2nd ed. Champaign, IL: Human Kinetics.

Loudon, J., S.L. Bell, and J.M. Johnston. 1998. *The clinical orthopedic assessment guide.* Champaign, IL: Human Kinetics.

Olds, T., and K. Norton. 1999. *Pre-exercise health screening guide.* Champaign, IL: Human Kinetics.

Whiting, W.C., and R.F. Zernicke. 1998. *Biomechanics of musculoskeletal injury.* Champaign, IL: Human Kinetics.

CHAPTER 9

Fitness Assessment

Gregory S. Anderson, PhD
Brian Justin, MHK

Key Terms

$\dot{V}O_2$max

submaximal test

rating of perceived exertion (RPE)

internal fat

bioelectric impedance analysis

standardization

muscular strength

muscular endurance

Review Questions

1. How could a fitness and lifestyle assessment help personal trainers serve their clients better?

   _____

   _____

2. In order to perform the active portions of a fitness assessment, clients should have a resting HR of _____ bpm, a systolic pressure that must not exceed _____ mmHg, and diastolic pressure that must not exceed _____ mmHg.

3. Describe proper exercise order.

   _____

   _____

4. True or false: The patterning of adipose tissue distribution is more important to health than the total amount of adipose tissue.

   _____

5. What are the drawbacks to using bioelectric impedance analysis for body composition?

   _____

   _____

6. Define *body mass index* and provide the range over which one would be considered to have low health risk.

   _____

   _____

7. A male who weighs 72 kilograms, is 174 centimetres tall, and has a waist girth of 104 centimetres would have a BMI of _____ and _____ relative risk of disease.

8. Grip strength is an example of what kind of strength test?

   _____

9. Describe the four sources of error in muscular fitness testing.

   _____

   _____

   _____

   _____

Multiple-Choice Questions

1. **Before testing clients should be told**
   a. to not exercise for 4 hours before
   b. to not drink alcohol for 1 hour before
   c. to not drink caffeine for 12 hours before
   d. all of the above

2. **Clients should not participate in the active portions of the fitness test if their resting**
   a. HR is greater than 100
   b. systolic BP is greater than 120
   c. diastolic BP is less than 75
   d. breathing rate is greater than 12 breaths per minute

3. **The tapping sounds heard when measuring BP are**
   a. Korotkoff sounds
   b. HR
   c. cardiac output
   d. pulse pressure

4. **An example of a test of muscular endurance is**
   a. completion of one chin-up
   b. repeated push-ups to exhaustion
   c. a grip strength test using a hand-grip dynamometer
   d. the vertical jump

5. **Prediction of $\dot{V}O_2$ max is dependent on measurement of**
   a. BP
   b. HR and workload
   c. height
   d. all of the above

References

Brooks, D. 2004. *The complete book of personal training.* Champaign, IL: Human Kinetics.

CSEP. 2003. *The Canadian physical activity, fitness, and lifestyle approach.* Ottawa, Ontario: Canadian Society for Exercise Physiology.

Heyward, V. 2006. *Advanced fitness assessment and exercise prescription,* 5th ed. Champaign IL: Human Kinetics.

Hoffman, J. 2006. *Norms for fitness, performance, and health.* Champaign, IL: Human Kinetics.

Niemen, D. 2007. *Exercise testing and prescription: A health related approach,* 6th ed. Dubuque, Iowa: McGraw Hill.

Program Design Concepts and Typical Personal Training Programs

Rod Macdonald, BEd

Key Terms

periodization

supercompensation

supercompression cycle

sum of training effect

progressive overload

specificity

Review Questions

1. **What are the four components of good program design?**

   _____

   _____

   _____

   _____

2. **What is the difference between open- and closed-chain exercises?**

   _____

   _____

3. **What are the key components of the first workout?**

   _____

   _____

4. **Outline the steps you should follow when making a program modification.**

   _____

   _____

   _____

   _____

5. **The best set performance if you are short on time and want to target two muscle groups consecutively would be a _____ .**

Multiple-Choice Questions

1. **The _____ is the largest component of a periodized program.**
   a. mesocycle
   b. macrocycle
   c. microcycle
   d. manocycle

2. **To apply periodization to program design, you must balance stress with**
   a. proper nutrition
   b. commitment
   c. recovery
   d. realistic goals

3. **You can train for as little as _____ of the volume but at the same intensity for up to 12 weeks to prevent reversibility.**
   a. 1/4
   b. 1/2
   c. 2/3
   d. 1/3

4. **An example of specificity as applied to marathon training would be**
   a. cycling to and from work Mondays, Wednesdays, and Fridays
   b. walking 10 to 15 minutes per day for 6 months
   c. running up and down stadium stairs
   d. progressively running longer distances for 12 to 24 weeks before the marathon

5. **After ceasing a regular workout routine of 3 days per week for 6 months, your client notices that muscle definition has begun to decrease. This is an example of**
   a. specificity
   b. recovery
   c. reversibility
   d. individualization

6. **Which of the following components is *not* important to gather before designing a program?**
   a. exercise history
   b. food intolerances
   c. client goals
   d. available equipment inventory

7. **If your client's goal is muscular development, where should strength training be positioned in relation to the program?**
   a. after the warm-up
   b. before the warm-up
   c. after the cardiorespiratory workout
   d. after the workout

8. **If you ask a client to perform an exercise with a tempo of 3:1:5:0, the *3* represents what?**
   a. the eccentric action of the movement
   b. the concentric action of the movement
   c. the pause between the eccentric and subsequent concentric action of the movement
   d. the pause between the concentric and subsequent eccentric action of the movement

9. **Which of the following is a disadvantage of working with free weights?**
   a. Free weights do not imitate real-world resistance.
   b. Free weights are relatively low cost.
   c. Free weights are sometimes hard to control.
   d. Free weights are versatile.

Short-Answer Questions

1. Describe the types of things you need to communicate to your clients about equipment that will permit them to work out on their own with confidence.

   _____

   _____

   _____

   _____

2. What are some of the elements you need to watch for with clients after the first few sessions?

   _____

   _____

   _____

   _____

References

American College of Sports Medicine. 2005. *ACSM's guidelines for exercise testing and prescription*, 7th ed. Philadelphia, PA: Lippincott, Williams and Wilkins.

Bompa, T.O. 1999. *Periodization: Theory and methodology of training*, 4th ed. Champaign, IL: Human Kinetics.

Brooks, D. 1998. *Program design for personal trainers: Bridging theory into application.* Champaign, IL: Human Kinetics.

National Strength and Conditioning Association. 2000. *Essentials of strength training and conditioning*, 2nd ed. Champaign, IL: Human Kinetics.

Wilmore, J.H., and D.L. Costill, 2004. *Physiology of sport and exercise*, 3rd ed. Champaign, IL: Human Kinetics.

Zaryski, C., and Smith, D.J. 2005. Training principles and issues for ultra-endurance athletes. *Current Sports Medicine Reports* 4: 165-170.

CHAPTER 12

Psychology of Personal Training

Mike Bates, MBA

Key Terms

behavior change

pre-contemplation

contemplation

preparation

action

maintenance

exercise adherence

SMART goals

lifestyle fitness coaching

Review Questions

1. List five qualities of an effective counselor in a personal training setting.

_____

_____

_____

_____

_____

2. Describe the five stages in the stages of change model.

_____

_____

_____

_____

_____

3. List five of the general motivational strategies.

_____

_____

_____

_____

_____

4. Describe how environmental factors play a key role in predicting the likelihood of someone's success on an exercise program.

_____

_____

_____

_____

5. Apply the SMART acronym to goals for a new exerciser who wants to lose weight.

_____

_____

_____

_____

6. List of five of the common beliefs and misconceptions that new exercisers have.

_____

_____

_____

_____

Multiple-Choice Questions

1. The cognitive variables that have been the best predictors of physical activity are _____ and _____.
   a. self-efficacy; self-reliance
   b. self-efficacy; self-motivation
   c. goal setting; experience
   d. goal setting; ability to focus

2. Studies have shown that women tend to prefer to exercise
   a. on their own
   b. in small groups
   c. with a partner
   d. in the water

3. The stages of change model is also known as the
   a. behaviour modification model
   b. transmyopic model
   c. transfat model
   d. transtheoretical model

4. During this stage, the client has started to think about exercising and has most likely identified a potential course of action.
   a. preparation
   b. action
   c. contemplation
   d. precontemplation

5. Self-monitoring and self-reinforcement are characteristics of what stage?
   a. preparation
   b. action
   c. contemplation
   d. precontemplation

References

Blair, S.N., A.L. Dunn, B.H. Marcus, R.A. Carpenter, and P. Jaret. 2001. *Active living every day.* Champaign, IL: Human Kinetics.

Gavin, J. 2005. *Lifestyle fitness coaching.* Champaign, IL: Human Kinetics.

Griffin, J.C. 2006. *Client-centered exercise prescription,* 2nd ed. Champaign, IL: Human Kinetics.

Howley, E.T., and B.D. Franks. 2003. *Health fitness instructor's handbook,* 4th ed. Champaign, IL: Human Kinetics.

Marcus, B.H., and L. Forsyth. 2003. *Motivating people to be physically active.* Champaign, IL: Human Kinetics.

Weinberg, R.S., and D. Gould. *Foundations of sport and exercise psychology,* 3rd ed. Champaign, IL: Human Kinetics.

CHAPTER 13

Business of Personal Training

Mike Bates, MBA

Key Terms

4 Ps of marketing

differentiation

isochrone

direct mail

guerrilla marketing

circle of influence

litigious situations

insurance

Review Questions

1. Describe the concept of differentiation and list four ways you can apply it to yourself.

   _____

   _____

   _____

   _____

2. List four different ways you can price your services as a personal trainer.

   _____

   _____

   _____

   _____

3. What are the key factors to consider when determining your pricing structure?

   _____

   _____

   _____

   _____

4. Why is it important to track where your new clients are coming from and how they are hearing about you?

   _____

   _____

   _____

   _____

5. List the seven steps you can follow when selling personal training.

   _____

   _____

   _____

   _____

   _____

6. What are the common objections you will get when you are trying to sell your services and how can you overcome them?

   _____

   _____

   _____

7. **List five things that are important for your professional image.**

    _____

    _____

    _____

    _____

    _____

8. **What are the main components of the personal training agreement?**

    _____

    _____

    _____

    _____

9. **Identify the potential litigious situations that personal trainers might encounter.**

    _____

    _____

    _____

    _____

10. **In the following chart, list two advantages and two disadvantages for each type of promotion.**

TYPE	ADVANTAGES	DISADVANTAGES
Direct mail		
Print ads		
Electronic media		
General networking		
Guerrilla marketing		
Media outreach		
Referrals		

11. What defines whether or not personal trainers are working for a club or themselves?

_____

_____

_____

_____

Multiple-Choice Questions

1. Which of the following is not one of the 4 Ps of marketing?
a. product
b. price
c. place
d. program

2. The isochrone is typically a travel radius of _____ minutes around your location.
a. 5 to 7
b. 8 to 12
c. 15 to 20
d. 20 to 30

3. _____ is the perception that people have about you and your business.
a. Positioning
b. Pricing
c. Differentiation
d. Marketing

4. The key to long-term success as a personal trainer is your ability to generate
a. traffic
b. phone calls
c. referrals
d. publicity

5. Asking "When can we get started?" is an example of which type of closing method?
a. trial close
b. alternate close
c. suggestive close
d. assumptive close

6. Which of the following is not an important part of the personal training agreement?
a. appointment time
b. fees
c. cancellation policy
d. informed consent

References

Mullin, B.J., S. Hardy, and W.A. Sutton. 1999. *Sport marketing*, 2nd ed. Champaign, IL: Human Kinetics.

CASE STUDIES

Use the following case studies to assist in preparing for the Theory and Practical exam. Use the sheets included in the exam preparation (cardiovascular and resistance training sheets) to assist in your response. Use chapters 10 and 11 of *Foundations of Professional Personal Training* to guide your work. The answers are not provided. Don't forget to also get some practice doing fitness assessments and creating programs with your friends, family and co-workers.

1. Jerry is a 20-year-old student and has hired you as his personal trainer. He gained 6.8 kg (15 pounds) in his first year of university and wants to improve his muscle tone as soon as possible. Jerry has a resting heart rate of 72 bpm and a resting blood pressure of 120/80 mmHg. His current body weight is 81.6 kg (180 pounds) and he is 175 cm (5 feet, 9 inches) tall. He likes to exercise and play sports, but has not really trained since the school year ended 4 months ago. The other information you collected for his fitness assessment is as follows:

- Waist circumference—28 cm
- Body fat % (from bioelectrcial impedance analysis)—24%
- Push-ups—20
- Curl-ups—23
- $\dot{V}O_2$max—38 millilitres per kilogram per minute
- Sit-and-reach—27 cm

2. Erin is a 45-year-old investment advisor who wants to increase her lean muscle mass as well as drop the 4.5 kg (10 pounds) she has gained from too many executive lunches. She is active with squash and golf in the summer and exercises at a fitness club once a week in the winter. Her resting heart rate is 65 bpm and her resting blood pressure is 125/82 mmHg. Her current body weight is 61.2 kg (135 pounds) and she is 160 cm (5 feet, 3 inches) tall. The other information you collected for her fitness assessment is as follows:

- Waist circumference—24 cm
- Body fat % (from bioelectrcial impedance analysis)—22%
- Push-ups—17
- Curl-ups—25
- $\dot{V}O_2$max—33 millilitres per kilogram per minute
- Sit-and-reach—30

ANSWERS TO MULTIPLE-CHOICE QUESTIONS

Chapter 1 Principles of Fitness, Health, and Wellness Concepts

1. a	5. a	8. c
2. d	6. c	9. a
3. d	7. b	10. d
4. b		

Chapter 2 Nutrition Concepts for Personal Trainers

1. d	6. c	11. c
2. b	7. b	12. a
3. c	8. d	13. c
4. c	9. a	14. d
5. a	10. c	15. d

Chapter 3 Bioenergetics Concepts

1. c	6. c	11. b
2. b	7. a	12. c
3. a	8. b	13. a
4. c	9. d	14. c
5. a	10. c	15. a

Chapter 4 Cardiorespiratory Concepts

1. d	6. d	11. d
2. a	7. a	12. d
3. d	8. d	13. b
4. a	9. c	14. c
5. d	10. b	

Chapter 5 Skeletal Anatomy and Flexibility Concepts

1. d	4. a
2. a	5. c
3. d	6. d

Chapter 6 Muscular Concepts

1. b	5. b	9. d
2. b	6. a	10. d
3. c	7. c	11. a
4. a	8. b	

Chapter 7 Injury Recognition Concepts

1. e	7. a	12. d
2. b	8. c	13. d
3. d	9. d	14. d
4. d	10. d	15. a
5. c	11. e	16. e
6. c		

Chapter 8 Preexercise Screening

1. a	3. d	5. c
2. c	4. d	

Chapter 9 Fitness Assessment

1. c	3. a	5. b
2. a	4. b	

Chapters 10 and 11 Program Design Concepts and Typical Personal Training Programs

1. b	4. d	7. a
2. c	5. c	8. b
3. d	6. b	9. c

Chapter 12 Psychology of Personal Training

1. b	3. d	5. b
2. a	4. c	

Chapter 13 Business of Personal Training

1. d	3. a	5. d
2. b	4. c	6. a

ABOUT CAN-FIT-PRO

Can-Fit-Pro, a division of Canadian Fitness Professionals, Inc., was established in 1993 to provide Canadian fitness professionals with continuing education and professional support. In 1998, Can-Fit-Pro launched its national certification program designed to provide one standardized, comprehensive certification body in Canada for specialists in fitness instruction, personal training, nutrition and wellness, program direction, and club management. Known for quality and enthusiasm, a Can-Fit-Pro certification establishes a benchmark for excellence and education in the fitness industry. Can-Fit-Pro's *Foundations of Professional Personal Training* is used by Can-Fit-Pro for their Personal Training Specialist certification program for candidates who work with clients on an individual basis and design exercise programs for improved health and fitness.

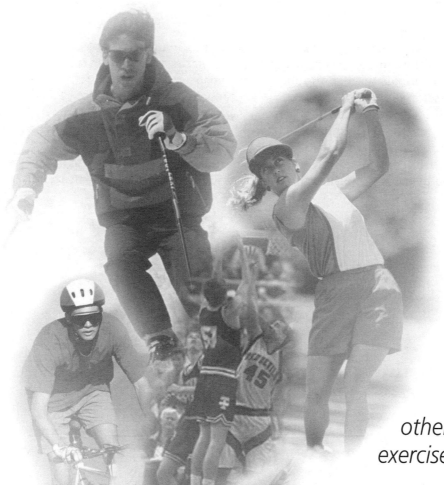